BREAST TO NORMAL CHEST

BREAST TO NORMAL CHEST

DR AMIT GUPTA

Worldwide Publishing by
Pendown Press

PENDOWN PRESS
An ISO 9001 & ISO 14001 Certified Co.,
Regd. Office: 2525/193, 1st Floor, Onkar Nagar-A, Tri Nagar, Delhi-110035
Ph.: 09350849407, 09312235086
E-mail: info@pendownpress.com
Branch Office: 1A/2A, 20, Hari Sadan, Ansari Road, Daryaganj, New Delhi-110002
Ph.: 011-45794768
Website: PendownPress.com

First Edition: 2023

ISBN: 978-93-5554-492-6

Layout and Cover Designed by Pendown Graphics Team
Printed and Bound in India by Thomson Press India Ltd.

CONTENTS

Chapter 1

Hello, Let's Get Acquainted

Hello, I am Dr Amit Gupta. Today, I am blessed to be counted among India's most influential Plastic Surgeons and my team today performs the largest number of Male breast reduction surgeries in India.

To date, my team at Divine Cosmetic Surgery has performed 5000+ Gynecomastia surgeries with unbelievable success.

This means that 5000+ people live a life of freedom, filled with confidence, without feeling abnormal, awkward or ashamed due to Gynecomastia.

We have created a new International Classification of Gynecomastia published in the Indian Journal of Plastic Surgery.

This classification will rock all current classifications and change the way that the world looks at Indian Plastic Surgeons. We now have the ability to stand shoulder-to-shoulder with the Best Medical Innovators in the world.

I am a Gold medallist from Maulana Azad Medical College and have done Fellowships in Plastic Surgery from Brazil and Belgium.

I founded DIVINE COSMETIC SURGERY in the year 2011 in the month of March with the sole intent of making the safest, state-of-the-art surgery options accessible and affordable to as many people as possible.

Thanks to the power and purity of our intent, slowly but surely, we have progressed to building our own hospital in the premium location of GK 2 in South Delhi.

By the grace of the almighty, this is the largest niche Plastic Surgery Center in the entire Northern part of India, which means we can serve more number of people.

Over the years, I have treated an extremely large number of patients suffering from Gynecomastia, and realised that standardisation in the treatment of male breast enlargement was missing.

This was leading to too many complications happening at the hands of younger doctors simply due to the basic concepts of treatment not being understood.

The whole new concept of Gynecomastia 360 4DX Framework is totally aimed at creating a standardised approach for every patient who wants treatment for male breast enlargement across the country and across the globe in a way that ensures near 100% safety and near 100% fail-safe procedure.

This new concept has the potential to completely disrupt the current practice of surgical treatment. In this book, I will share in detail why this whole concept was created, and the finer details of this concept will be discussed.

I am immensely thankful to my team of Plastic Surgeons, our surgical assistants, our consultants who interact with the patients, and my digital creation team, who are responsible for creating beautiful and educational videos and bringing my thoughts to real life.

Chapter 2

How It All Began

So, you might be wondering, how did my love for treating Gynecomastia begin?

Initially, I had no special attachment or favoritism toward the treatment of Gynecomastia. This specific treatment was just another form of treatment in the entire repertoire of Plastic surgery treatments that I used to offer to my patients. On average such surgeries used to be around 5 or 6 a month.

Regrettably, at that time, I never looked at it in depth. I hardly ever interacted with any patient to understand why they wanted to undergo such treatment or really assess their need for it. I just finished the procedure to the best of my ability as a Surgeon, saw the happy faces, and that was the end of it.

However, things changed completely one day. On that momentous day, a patient who was older than me was being prepared for an aesthesiain the main operating theatre.

Upon seeing me, he immediately got up from the table and touched my feet. I was genuinely taken aback and, in fact, even embarrassed.

I shyly asked him why he did this, and his response truly startled me and shook me up. He said that I was God for him that day and was blessing him with a new life.

I was totally shaken because, for me, till that day, it was just another surgery.

Till then, I had no idea of the impact my surgeries were having on people's lives and well-being.

That day proved to be a turning point, and following that day, I started interacting with every patient who was undergoing this surgery, and I made sure to understand and take t note of why they were undergoing this surgery and what would be the importance of this procedure in their life.

The results of these interactive discussions were Earth shattering for me. And for the first time, **I realised the real importance of this surgery and the amount of confidence I was giving back to each patient because of my actions.**

I was shocked and saddened to learn that patients suffering from Gynecomastia had very low self-esteem, and they did not feel free to wear certain clothes that highlighted their condition.

Also, they felt that their relationships were not as great as they wanted them to be due to society's judgements and their own insecurities.

Teenagers were perhaps the worst affected as it is already a socially and emotionally awkward phase of life, which was compounded by this condition.

Many were unwilling to take up sports because they were embarrassed to be seen with large breasts, and many became introverts and started hiding from other students for fear of being ridiculed, singled out and bullied.

For some, things were so bad they even contemplated suicide.

This knowledge completely changed me from the inside and changed the way I started interacting with and sending messages to patients suffering from this problem.

For me now, it was no longer about surgery only, it was a mission, and this mission was to successfully treat each and every patient suffering from Gynecomastia in the safest possible mechanism and to give them back their life and their confidence.

That day I made a decision to personally involve myself with every patient and hand hold them till their entire recovery and watch them smile as they developed the confidence to wear the clothes of their choice and fulfill the dreams and goals they aimed for in life.

We worked hard to find better solutions, and the procedure for skin sagging was handled by creating the concept of a 'U' lift. For this, we worked on fixing the nipple by removing some skin from above the areola in a U pattern. This allowed us to fix the nipple to prevent further sagging of the skin.

It took me nearly 6 years to improve each step of this procedure in order to create this whole new concept of Gynecomastia 360 4Dx approach.

In this process, I faced a lot of resistance, even from my own team, because I was creating new concepts that were going against the established principles, and they feared that I might actually end up causing more problems.

But I persevered because I had the confidence that each and every step that I was creating was scientific. Also, it was just pure confidence in my own abilities and my desire to create something of value for Gynecomastia patients that allowed me to create this whole new concept.

This is something that is being really sought by each and every patient today who comes and consults us. We are proud and humbled at the same time to say that today we perform the largest number of Gynecomastia surgeries in the country.

My team and I have performed more than 5000 surgeries in the last 16 years, treating patients from not only India but across the globe from countries such as the USA, Australia, New Zealand, DUBAI, UK, Peru etc., to name a few.

Over the last 6 months alone, we have performed more than 100 surgeries using this new concept, and the results are absolutely outstanding.

Mr Piyush from Dubai underwent this procedure in Mayr, and this is what he has to say.

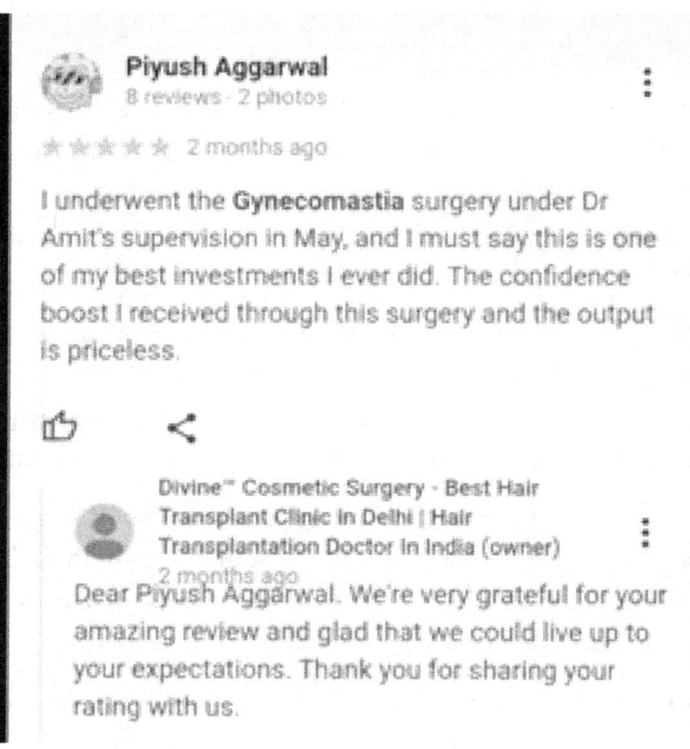

Mr Ajay added how his life has changed after this surgery.

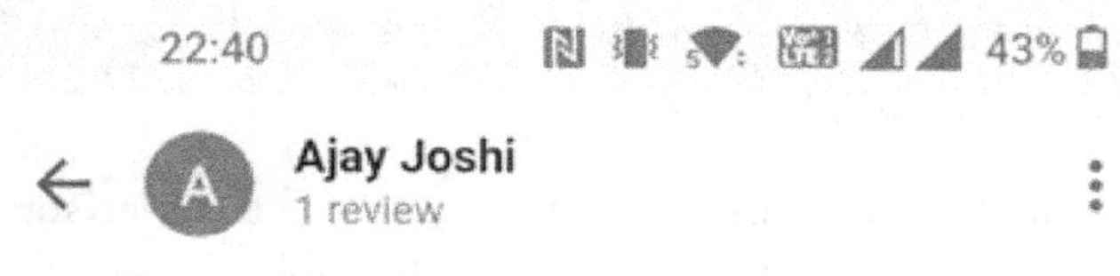

was facing gynaecimastia problem I can't got outside without shirt even in sweeming pool. I Checked online then I get know about **gynaecomastia** and knie about Dr Amiy Gupta I cansult him and he advised me for surgeeh itsbinly one day process next day bendage then I start my normal routine work and now 9 month done my life in on normal track and I can do what I want whenever I have any doubt Satpal give appointment and solve the problen thanx sir

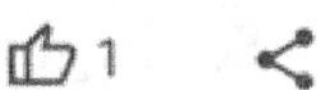

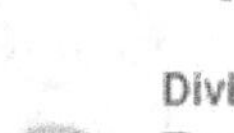

Divine™ Cosmetic Surgery - Best Hair Transplant Clinic in Delhi | Hair Transplantation Doctor In India (owner)

a month ago

Dear Ajay Joshi. We're very grateful for your amazing review and glad that we could live up to your expectations. Thank you for sharing your rating with us.

The biggest challenge we are facing in this industry is that, for some reason, new r Plastic Surgeons are not motivated enough r to undergo rigorous training and learn the finer details of managing Gynecomastia.

Due to this, the complication rates or the dissatisfaction grades of patients undergoing this procedure are very high, and a very large percentage of them seek revision procedures which add to their financial burden and economic burden because of the time away from their workplace.

As one of the most experienced teams in the country, we consider it our responsibility to create a solution because the onus lies with us.

To bridge this gap, we have created a Framework that can be easily followed by the Plastic Surgeons of the entire country.

And the proof that we have succeeded in our endeavor is evident in our delighted patients, who are overwhelmingly giving us testimonials, not only in writing but also on video.

These testimonials are being posted all across various social media platforms giving a huge amount of confidence to every new patient who wants to go through this procedure

My promise is that this new concept of "Gynecomastia 360 4Dx Framework" will completely revolutionise the way we perform such surgeries in this country and we foresee a near future where t every Plastic Surgeon in this country follows this concept in order to create better and better results.

I am today on a mission to treat every patient who is suffering from low confidence and lack of self-esteem due to male best enlargement in a way that is safer than before and has the fastest return to normal activity.

It is my invitation to every patient who is reading this to utilise this opportunity to change your life in the fastest manner possible because today, you have the option of y the most revolutionary and modern technique performed by the most experienced Gynecomastia Surgeon in the country. Don't let this opportunity of living a life of freedom pass you by!

Chapter 3

Why this Book?

Many might be wondering why I am writing this book. Well, the answer is simple:

"Because I am creating Trust with my Care philosophy."

Today, my team and I work intensively with each and every Gynecomastia patient to understand their problems and the solution that they are looking for. Then we present them with this new concept and explain to them that this is not being offered to them by any other Plastic surgery team in the entire country. And then, we go on to showcase the benefits of this new concept.

There were many problems arising out of surgeries for Gynecomastia, and the most common problems why we decided to create this new concept were:

1. Damage to the nipple area in many

2. Asymmetry

3. Lack of attention to sagging of the breast

4. Not handling fat in the axilla and side rolls

5. Creating depression in the 6 O clock position of the chest 6. Creating dish or depressed nipple deformity

6. Seeing bad scars

7. Incomplete removal of fat

8. Seeing caved-in or flat chest deformity

My dream for all the Plastic Surgeons operating on Gynecomastia patients is that they provide the perfect results by preventing the above-stated 9 problems.

By preventing these issues, we are automatically creating the most brilliant results, increasing the trust and confidence of our patients in the Plastic Surgery Fraternity.

However, it is essential that each and every Plastic Surgeon must also train themselves in this new technique in order to recreate the success that we are creating.

With this book, we aim to reach out to each and every male who is embarrassed by his male chest problem.

We want to reach out to them and tell them that:

1. You are now safer than ever

2. You can now expect fail safe results

3. Your chances of complications are now reduced dramatically

4. You will get the maximum confidence that will last your lifetime

5. You can wear the clothes of your dreams

6. You can build the body of your dreams

This book is the ONLY book in the world that understands you and talks about you, a person who is less confident about your looks and then goes on to offer a solution to your concerns. .

This is the only book that talks about Gynecomastia 360 4DX Framework, which is the new revolution in Gynecomastia treatment.

This is the only book that trains other Plastic Surgeons in this unique skill.

These are secrets that have taken us years to create, and we are sharing these with the world today to benefit each and every one of you.

This book is my gift of confidence to every male stopping himself from living a full life.

Chapter 4

What is the Concept of the Gynecomastia 360 4DX Framework?

Since our conversation through this book began, I have been talking about the safe and fail safe concept of the Gynecomastia 360 4DX Framework. Now let's understand it in more detail in this chapter. I am listing below each step of this revolutionary framework.

1. Use of VASER technology to emulsify the fat to make liposuction easier.

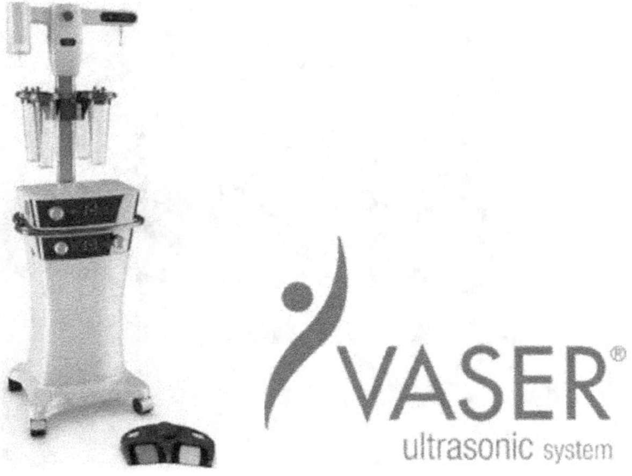

2. **Dividing the chest into grids** - the breast, axillary tail, axillary tyres, the inner lower quadrant and the upper inner quadrant of the breast.

3. **Defining the incisions** - in the areola and in the axilla.

4. **4DX or the 4 Direction Approach**

   a. Antegrade liposuction from the axilla to remove fat from the breast.

   b. Side liposuction from the areola to remove the axillary tyre.

   c. Opposite side liposuction of the infra areolar breast from the areola incision.

   d. Retrograde liposuction of the axillary tail

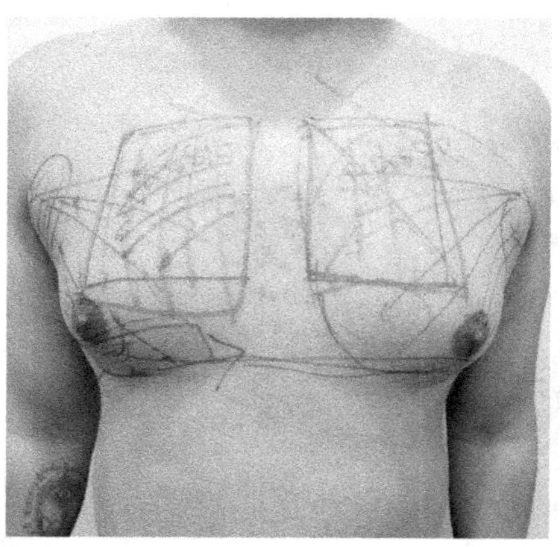

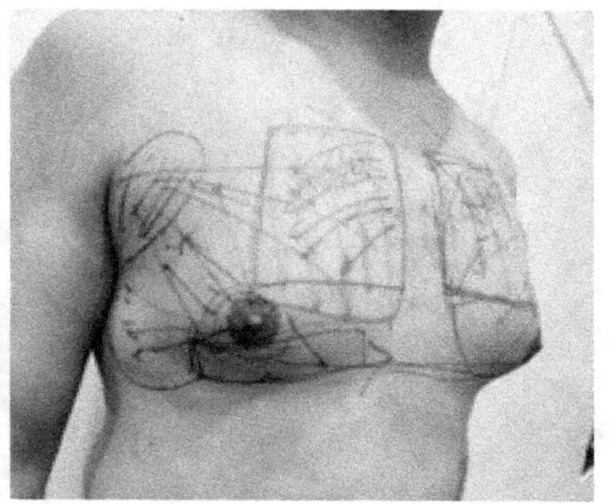

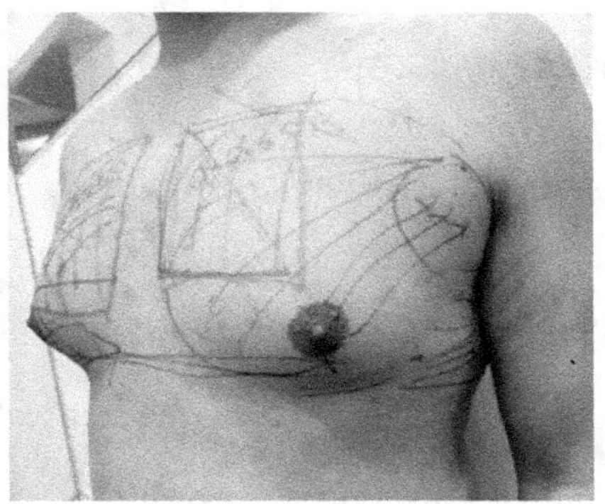

5. **No GO Zone** - This is the red box marked in the picture. Never perform liposuction in this zone. This avoids damage to the blood supply of the nipple without affecting the result.

6. **Nipple lift** in case of breast sagging.

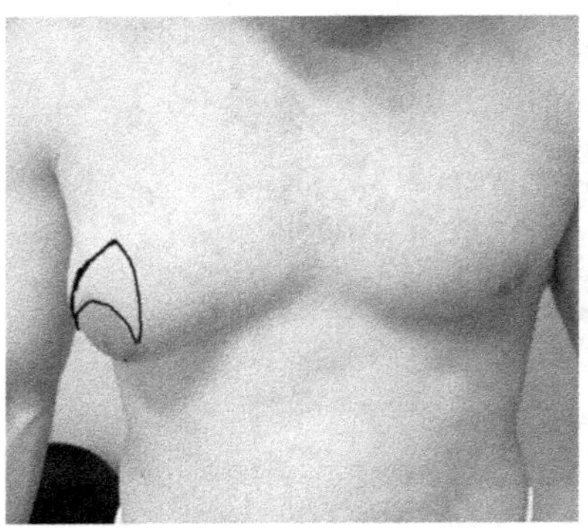

What is the 4DXFramework?

The 4DX Framework refers to the use of 4 different directions to tackle the 4 different regions of the chest. The benefits of this are:

1. No depression below the areola.

2. No depression in the lower quadrant of the breast.

3. Tackling the side tyre effectively.

4. Tackling fat in the axilla region (axillary tail) more effectively. This is mostly ignored by the majority of Plastic Surgeons,

What are the Important Landmarks of the Chest?

1. **The incision site**

    a.   from 5 to 7 o clock on the areola.

    b.   5 mm just behind the axilla.

2. **The Axillary Tail** - the area on the side of the breast just touching the axilla.

3. **The Axillary Tyre** - the bulge by the side of the breast below the axilla.

4. **The Upper Inner Quadrant** - NO TOUCH ZONE

5. **The Lower Inner Quadrant** - Ensure that you take out all fat completely.

What is the Sequence of the Steps of the Gynecomastia 360 4DXFramework?

1. Marking of the chest to define the grids.

2. Infiltration of the saline solution.

3. Use of Vaser.

4. Liposuction using the 4DXFramework.

5. Gland-sparing gland removal - leaving behind 5-8 percent of the gland to prevent nipple depression.

6. Scarless suturing - using the internal buttress stitch to prevent scarring.

Chapter 5

The 7 Key Steps to Ensure a Perfect Result in Gynecomastia Surgery

Now that you are aware of the steps, their details and their sequence, here are a few critical points that you need to take care of to get perfect results from your Gynecomastia surgery.

1. **Ensure adequate and not over infiltration** – we suggest a maximum amount of local anaesthesia infiltration as per grade.

    a. We usually advise 1:1 infiltration (1 ml infiltration for every 1 ml fat aspiration expected).

Grade	Amount of fluid infiltration (each side) in ml
1a	100
1b	150-200
2a	250 - 500
2b	250-500
3a	750 - 1000
3b	750 - 1000
4a	1000 - 1500 ml

    b. This prevents subsequent seroma formation.

2. **No over-suctioning** – always leave some amount of fat in the chest, and do not attempt to take all of it away. Leaving a thin layer of fat over the muscle and under the skin gives the appearance of a normal, not operated chest.

   The telltale signs of an operated chest are:

   a. A depressed nipple

   b. An asymmetric chest

   c. Deformations in the chest

   d. A badly placed incision

   e. Loss of nipple

   f. Loss of areola

3. **Invisible incisions** – incision for liposuction should be hidden in the axillary fold, and the incision for gland removal to be made at the junction of the areola and skin. This makes the incision virtually invisible.

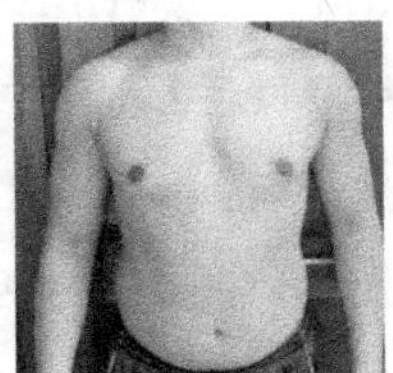 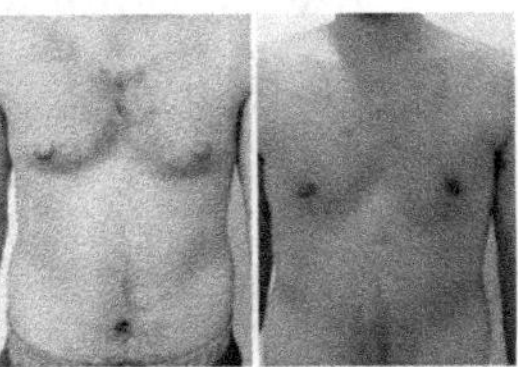 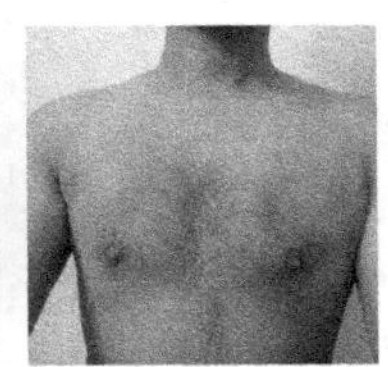

4. **Always leave 2 to 3 mm of gland tissue below the areola to maintain the shape of the areola.** Failure to do so will leave a deformity called "dish deformity" (as shown in the picture below). This is very ugly and gives the appearance of being operated on.

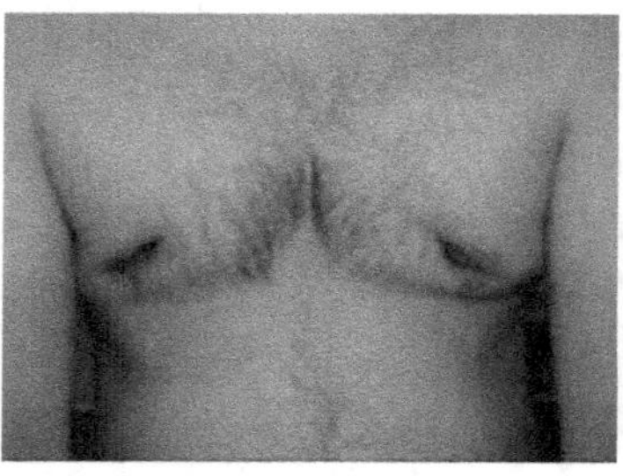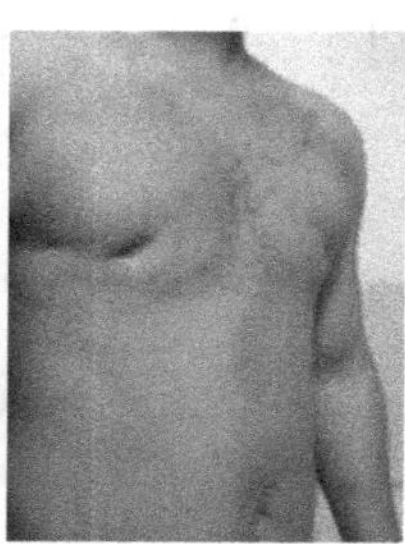

5. **Never excise tissue from inferior to the nipple –** Only perform liposuction; any excision of the tissue only leads to bad depression deformity.

6. **Getting a good, virtually scarless suture –** a great suture is achieved by 2means

    a. Internal buttress suture – placing a stich between gland below the nipple and the dermis of the skin crease, allows a buttress for the areola, preventing any deformity.

    b. Fine sutures in a A stich form – suture is taken from the areola side, passing in a subcuticular fashion from the lower skin incision and back to the areola.

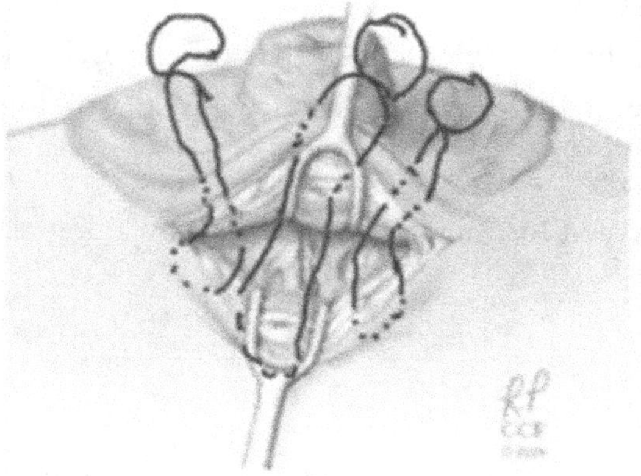

7. **Pressure bandaging** - use of elastic compression for 24 hours, followed by pressure garment for 3 weeks, is mandatory to get the desired results.

Addendum

We are delighted to add here that our new classification has been accepted by the Indian Journal of Plastic Surgery.

Over the last 16 years, we have worked very hard to collect data and then formulate the new path-breaking classification.

Table 1- New Proposed Gynecomastia Classification

Grade	Description of Grade	Explanation	Infiltration volume + Treatment Plan
1a	Puffy Nipple	No obvious problem visible except stretched areola with a button type feel	50ml + Excision in LA from intra areolar incision
1b	Minor breast enlargement	The breast is visibly bigger, limited fat, 250 ml with higher amount of fibroglandular tissue	200ml + Suction and gland excision in LA from intra areolar incision and stab in the inframammary area
2a	Moderate breast enlargement	The fat component is between 250-500gm. No ptosis expected	500ml + Suction- stab incision in axillary area and gland excision in GA from the intra areolar incision
2b	Moderate breast enlargement with ptosis	The fat component is between 250-500gm. Large gland components in the form of a conical breast. U lift needed for ptosis.	500ml + Suction from stab incision in axillary area & gland excision + U skin lift from supra areolar approach in GA
3a	Large chest enlargement with side rolls without ptosis	Chest is enlarged. Fat component is 500-750gm. Fat in breast rolls. No ptosis expected.	1000ml (each side and axilla) + Suction from stab incision in axillary area & gland excision h in GA
3b	Large Severe chest enlargement with side rolls with ptosis expected	Chest is enlarged, fat component + axilla rolls + ptosis expected/present	1000ml (each side and axilla) + Suction from stab incision in axillary area & gland excision + U skin lift from supra areolar approach in GA
4a	Severe chest enlargement without significant ptosis	Chest is severely enlarged. >750gm fat component + axilla rolls without significant ptosis. No need for skin lift	1500 ml (each side and axilla) + Suction from stab incision in axillary area & gland excision h in GA
4b	Severe chest enlargement with significant ptosis.	Chest is very big, huge breast rolls. significant ptosis requiring skin lift procedure	1500 ml (each side and axilla) + Suction from stab incision in axillary area & gland excision + U skin lift from supra areolar approach in GA. 2nd stage O lift (circumferential skin mastopexy may be needed. May need 2nd stage for tackling excess skin or same stage axillary roles excision

Chapter 6

This Condition Deserves A Solution

To be able to clearly illustrate what we are trying to solve here and what the challenges we are taking care of, let me share with you a small story in this chapter.

We were consulted by a 29-year-old male suffering from very low esteem. He was not able to progress in his job or wear the clothes of his choice. Even in the gym, he would wear loose-fitting clothes to hide his condition. In addition, his relationship with women was never perfect. It affected him emotionally and sexually both. He always hesitated during sexual activity due to his feeling of embarrassment at having large breasts. Life was difficult and frustrating for him on all counts.

We planned and performed a Gynecomastia 360 4 DX Framework procedure for him.

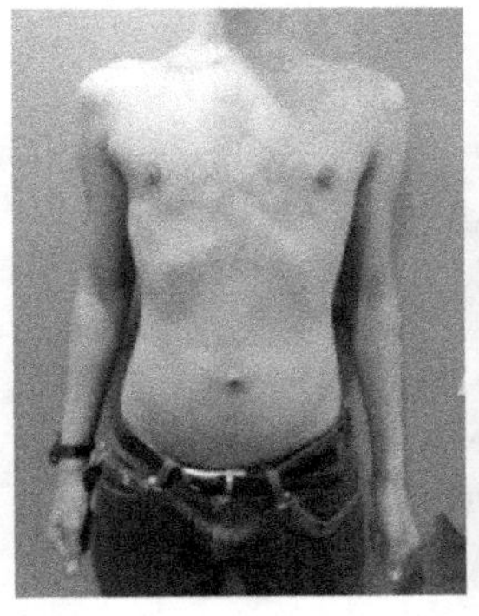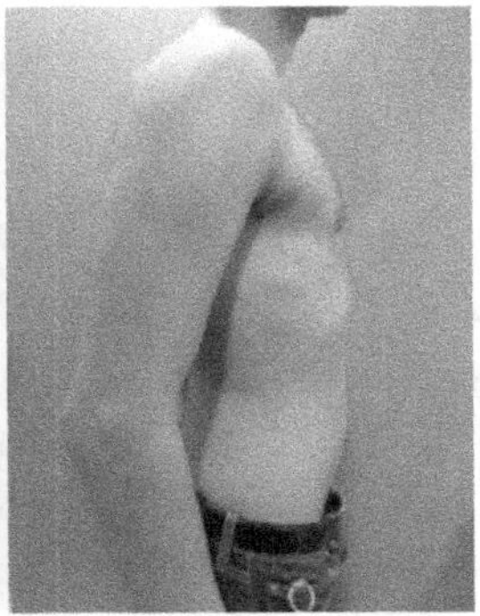

In as soon as 7 days, his entire persona changed.

His clothing changed to tight t-shirts. He said he felt more confident in the gym and while meeting colleagues at work.

His family came and hugged me and said their son had changed completely in just 7 days, and they wished he had done the procedure sooner.

With this approach, we will permanently solve the following:

1. Lowest chances of complications.

2. Reduced seroma.

3. Symmetric shapes.

4. Complete chest and not just breast reshaping.

5. Return to office in as soon as 1 day.

6. Discharge from the hospital within 4 hours

Chapter 7

What do our Patients say about us?

The success of this transformational framework is evident in the overwhelming and heart-warming testimonials from our delighted patients.

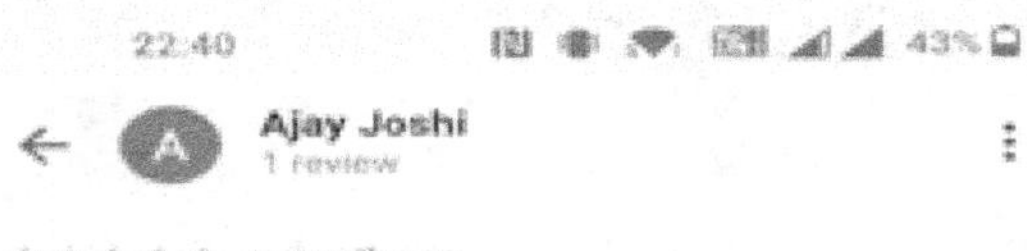

22:40   43%

← Tarun Kumar
1 review

★★★★★ 2 months ago

I had very fat deposit in my chest. Inspite of regular workout and diet it was not going fully i lost weight but not fat from chest. I got information from internet about **gynaecomastia** and I got to know about Dr Amit Gupta after one video consultation took appointment for my final discuss about surgery Dr Amit explain me everything and I can start my normal routine work from next days. Until the surgery and discharge everything was well taken care. Everything was smooth weather surgery and post care shivam explain all pre instructions and Mr satpal meet after the surgery explain about my all query and they call and insure all going good Or not. He is alaway responsive weather its working day Or holiday. Now after three month done of my surgery I cant even see my surgery scar . Thanx sir.

Divine™ Cosmetic Surgery - Best Hair Transplant Clinic in Delhi | Hair Transplantation Doctor In India (owner)
2 months ago
Dear Tarun Kumar. We're very grateful for your amazing review and glad that we could live up to your expectations. Thank you for sharing your rating with us.

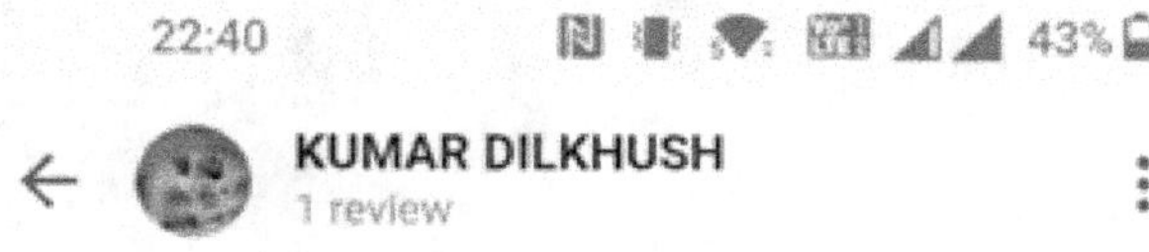

22:40

KUMAR DILKHUSH
1 review

★★★★★ 2 months ago

Dr.Amit Gupta is the best Plastic surgeon in Delhi.All Staff is best behaviour.I don't know all Members name but Shivam Bhaiya and Satpal Je is the Best Consultant and Help me.Without their help, My **Gynecomastia** surgery was not possible. I bow down to everyone, especially Amit sir, Shivam Bhaiya and Satpal Bhaiya.Thank you so much to all of you for influencing my life and giving me a new life. Thank you All Members in Devine Cosmetic surgery.😔😔🖤🖤🖤🖤🙏🙏🙏 😔Nitesh 😔

Divine™ Cosmetic Surgery - Best Hair Transplant Clinic in Delhi | Hair Transplantation Doctor In India (owner)
2 months ago
Dear DILKHUSH Kumar. We're very grateful for your amazing review and glad that we could live up to your expectations. Thank you for sharing your rating with us.

What Next?

As a patient suffering from Male Breast Enlargement (Gynecomastia), I would like to congratulate you for being aware of your problem and showing a willingness to change.

With this entire New Concept that will disrupt the way Gynecomastia surgery will be done in India, we invite you to experience this whole concept starting with a consultation with me.

I have developed this new framework, and I promise you that we will partner with you all the way to ensure that you get amazing confidence and highly enhanced self-esteem once again.

We promise that you will progress faster in your professional life, do better in your personal life and be able to work out to get the body of your dreams. You will wear the clothes of your choice and have the ability to take off your shirt when you desire, such as at beaches, swimming pools and other outdoor activities.

How?? I am sure this is no longer the question you are posing to yourself.

Now that you have read the book, you have the new found confidence that everything will be great again with the Gynecomastia 360 4Dx Framework.

We look forward to seeing you take a step toward your new life of confidence and freedom at our New Hospital in GK2, Delhi.

Call 9811994417 to book an appointment or mail us at

info@divinecosmeticsurgery.com